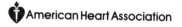
American Heart Association

Cholesterol Education Program
CLINICIAN'S
MANUAL
1991

D1473137

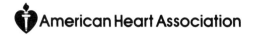
American Heart Association

Cholesterol Education Program

CLINICIAN'S MANUAL

1991

AM Gotto
The Methodist Hospital,
Baylor College of Medicine,
Houston, Texas, USA

Editorial Board
LA Carlson
King Gustav V Research Institute,
Stockholm, Sweden

DR Illingworth
The Oregon Health Sciences University,
Portland, Oregon, USA

GR Thompson
Hammersmith Hospital,
London, UK

△ **SANDOZ**

Developed in conjunction with the American Heart Association, the International Atherosclerosis Society, and Sandoz Pharmaceuticals Corporation.

ISSN 0961-7787
ISBN 1-870026-72-1

Foreword

After almost a century of advancement in our understanding of the risks of hyperlipidemia, the rationale for treating hyperlipidemia can no longer be questioned.

Early experimental studies showed that cholesterol is an important component of atherosclerotic plaques, and that the cholesterol found in these plaques entered them from the circulation. Clinical studies of families with premature atherosclerosis demonstrated in many cases inherited defects of cholesterol metabolism that resulted in very high levels of cholesterol in the blood. Prospective epidemiological trials such as the Framingham Heart Study have confirmed that high cholesterol levels are associated with heart disease.

Thus hypercholesterolemia, along with smoking and hypertension, has come to be recognized as one of the major risk factors for the development of atherosclerosis, the primary cause of coronary heart disease (CHD).

It has been accepted since 1963 that smoking cessation can reduce the risk of developing CHD; in the 1970s, the cardiovascular benefits of treating hypertension were established. In the 1980s, it became abundantly clear that lowering cholesterol levels (and, more specifically, lowering LDL-cholesterol levels) can slow or reverse the development of atherosclerosis and can reduce morbidity and mortality from CHD.

The evidence provided by these trials is incontrovertible. The question now is not whether high blood cholesterol levels should be treated, but rather when, in whom, and how. This *Manual* has therefore been designed to provide to clinicians information that is essential to the understanding and management of hyperlipidemia.

Robert I. Levy, MD
President, Sandoz Research Institute

Contents

Acknowledgments

Page 3. Adapted with permission from Martin *et al. Lancet* 1986;ii:933–936.

Page 4. Adapted with permission from *MKSAP VII.* Philadelphia: American College of Physicians, 1986.

Page 7. Adapted with permission from Thompson. *A Handbook of Hyperlipidaemia.* London: Current Science, 1989.

Page 11. (Top) Adapted with permission from Schonfeld. *Artery* 1979;5:305–329.

Page 11. (Bottom) Data from Lipid Research Clinics Program. *Circulation* 1979;60:427–439.

Page 12. Adapted with permission from Brown and Goldstein. *Science* 1986, 232:34–47. © The Nobel Foundation, 1986.

Page 18. Adapted with permission from Howard. *J Lipid Res* 1987;28: 613–628.

Page 20. Adapted with permission from Martin *et al. Lancet* 1986;ii:933–936.

Page 21. (Top) Adapted from Keys. *Circulation* 1970;51(suppl I):I-186–I-195, with permission of the American Heart Association, Inc.

Page 21. (Bottom) Adapted with permission from Kannel. *J Cardiovasc Pharmacol* 1989;13(suppl I):S4–S10.

Pages 22–23. Adapted with permission from Thompson. *A Handbook of Hyperlipidaemia.* London: Current Science, 1989.

Page 24. Published by courtesy of Professor M. Davies.

Page 25. Data from Brensike *et al. Circulation* 1984;69:313–324; Blankenhorn *et al. JAMA* 1987;257:3233–3240; Brown *et al. Circulation* 1989;80 (suppl II):266 (abstract).

Page 28. Adapted with permission from Thompson. In *Biochemical Aspects of Human Disease,* edited by Elkeles and Tavill. Oxford: Blackwell, 1983, pp 85–123.

Page 31. Adapted with permission from Report of the National Cholesterol Education Program Expert Panel. *Arch Intern Med* 1988;148:36–69.

Page 42. Adapted with permission from Report of the National Cholesterol Education Program Expert Panel. *Arch Intern Med* 1988;148:36–69.

Page 44. Adapted with permission from Report of the National Cholesterol Education Program Expert Panel. *Arch Intern Med* 1988;148:36–69.

Page 45. Adapted with permission from Report of the National Cholesterol Education Program Expert Panel. *Arch Intern Med* 1988;148:36–69.

Introduction

Americans are now keenly aware of the need to control hypercholesterolemia and other lipid disorders as a means of preventing coronary heart disease (CHD). Media health reports and food product advertisements have helped to bring the cholesterol–coronary disease connection to the forefront of patients' concerns. However, for many clinicians, this heightened patient awareness has not yet resulted in a more aggressive management of hyperlipidemia.

One problem, according to a survey conducted in 1989 by the US National Center for Health Statistics [1], is that clinicians still feel inadequately prepared to handle both the diagnosis of hyperlipidemia and its dietary and pharmaceutical management.

This uncertainty exists despite efforts toward educating clinicians by the National Institutes of Health (NIH), through its National Cholesterol Education Program (NCEP) [2] and by the American Heart Association (AHA), through its Physician Education Program.

It is hoped that the publication of this *Clinician's Manual* will help to answer the questions clinicians may still have regarding hyperlipidemia and its management. An attempt has been made to present the material in the *Manual* in a simple, straightforward manner. I believe that it represents a comprehensive approach toward antihyperlipidemic treatment. I hope that the *Manual* will help clinicians to be more effective in the diagnosis of hyperlipidemia and in its treatment. The *Manual* should also help clinicians to determine the potential benefits and possible side effects of dietary or drug intervention. In the long run, if the *Manual* is useful to clinicians, their patients will be better served.

I am grateful to Caroline Black of Current Science and to my editor, Anita Cecchin, for their outstanding assistance. I am also grateful to Sandoz Pharmaceuticals for its sponsorship of this edition.

Antonio M. Gotto Jr, MD, DPhil

1 What is hyperlipidemia and why should it be treated?

DEFINITION
Hyperlipidemia is present when serum lipids (**cholesterol** or **triglycerides**, or both) reach levels associated with increased risk of CHD.

The NCEP has categorized a patient's CHD risk on the basis of his or her total and low-density-lipoprotein (LDL) cholesterol levels, and the NIH 1984 Consensus Conference on Hypertriglyceridemia has established criteria for triglyceride values [3].

Lipid levels and CHD risk			
	Desirable	Borderline–high	High
Total cholesterol	< 200 mg/dL	200–239 mg/dL	≥ 240 mg/dL
LDL cholesterol	< 130 mg/dL	130–159 mg/dL	≥ 160 mg/dL
Triglycerides	< 250 mg/dL	250–500 mg/dL	> 500 mg/dL

These values must be viewed as arbitrary, and one should think more in terms of ranges than absolute values. Furthermore, the relationship between triglycerides and CHD risk is less clear than the relationship between total or LDL cholesterol and CHD risk. However, some hypertriglyceridemic patients, such as those with low high-density-lipoprotein (HDL) levels, are thought to be at increased risk for CHD.

The clinician should remember that the relationship between cholesterol levels and CHD is a continuous one. For example, data from the Multiple Risk Factor Intervention Trial (MRFIT) indicated that the rate of CHD increases continuously as patients' total cholesterol levels rise [4]. The relationship with total mortality was more complex, having a 'J-shaped' appearance. Thus, the cut-off points between

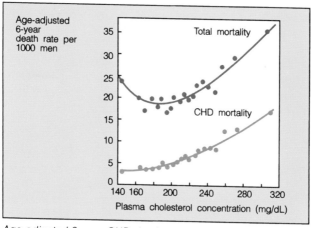

Age-adjusted 6-year CHD death rate per 1000 men screened for MRFIT according to serum cholesterol levels.

desirable, borderline, and high-risk cholesterol levels set by the NCEP are more arbitrary than they initially appear in the NCEP tables.

▶ *The clinician should always use his or her medical judgment and consider the patient's overall health when determining the most appropriate treatment.*

RATIONALE FOR TREATMENT

The level of cholesterol in the plasma is a major determinant of CHD in healthy people (see Section 7, *Lipids and cardiovascular risk*). Specifically, there is a direct correlation between CHD risk and concentrations of total or LDL cholesterol and an inverse correlation between risk and HDL cholesterol levels. Moreover, in the absence of hypercholesterolemia, the significance of the two other major modifiable risk factors — **smoking** and **hypertension** — declines significantly.

The primary treatment goal, therefore, is the reduction of total and LDL cholesterol levels, and, consequently, the risk of atherosclerosis and CHD. The evidence that lowering lipid concentrations to safe levels reduces the risk of coronary events is summarized in Section 7. Hypertriglyceridemia should be taken into consideration, depending on the particular clinical circumstances.

2 Classification of hyperlipidemia

LIPOPROTEIN PHENOTYPING

Cholesterol and triglyceride are transported through plasma by **lipoproteins** (see Section 3, *Lipids and lipoproteins*); **hypercholesterolemia** and **hypertriglyceridemia** reflect abnormalities in lipoprotein metabolism.

Fredrickson *et al.* divided the hyperlipidemias into six classes according to lipoprotein levels. **Lipoprotein phenotyping** distinguishes abnormalities involving increased LDL levels (leading to hypercholesterolemia) from those involving increased very-low-density-lipoprotein (VLDL) levels (leading to hypertriglyceridemia). Type I (hyperchylomicronemia) is extremely rare.

Note: This classification does not differentiate primary from secondary hyperlipidemias, and the lipoprotein phenotype of a hyperlipidemic individual can alter as a result of body-weight changes or treatment.

Classification of hyperlipoproteinemias			
Type	**Lipoprotein**	**Elevated lipid**	**Incidence (%)***
I	Chylo	TG	< 1
IIa	LDL	Chol	10
IIb	LDL + VLDL	TG + chol	40
III	IDL	TG + chol	< 1
IV	VLDL	TG ($\pm$ chol)	45
V	VLDL + chylo	TG ($\pm$ chol)	5

Chylo, chylomicrons; TG, triglyceride; chol, cholesterol.
*Percentage of patients with elevated lipid levels in USA.

Although it is often possible to classify the hyperlipidemias according to causative genetic defects, classifying them according to phenotype is useful as a guide to therapy.

TYPES OF HYPERLIPIDEMIA

The hyperlipidemias are heterogeneous and can be *primary*, i.e., due to genetic defects, or *secondary*, i.e., due to a number of metabolic, hormonal, or other disorders.

Major primary hyperlipidemias	Phenotype	Clinical disorders associated with secondary hyperlipidemia
Hypercholesterolemia		
Familial hypercholesterolemia

Polygenic hypercholesterolemia | IIa | Hypothyroidism
Nephrotic syndrome
Liver disease
Anorexia nervosa
Dysproteinemias |
| Mixed hyperlipidemias | | |
| Familial combined hyperlipidemias

Familial dysbetalipoproteinemia | IIb, IV, V

III | Hypothyroidism
Diabetes
Obesity
Anorexia nervosa
Liver disease |
| Hypertriglyceridemia | | |
| Familial hypertriglyceridemia | V, IV | Diabetes
Chronic renal disease
Alcohol
Diuretics
Beta blockers
Oral contraceptives |
| See Section 5, *Primary hyperlipidemia* | | See Section 6, *Causes of secondary hyperlipidemia* |

3 Lipids and lipoproteins

LIPIDS

The lipids **cholesterol** and **triglyceride** have important cellular functions: triglyceride is an energy source and cholesterol is a component of cell membranes; it is also a precursor of steroid hormones and bile acids. Since cholesterol in its esterified form and triglyceride are non-polar, they must be transported to their destinations by **lipoproteins**.

LIPOPROTEINS

Lipoproteins are spherical particles whose cores contain cholesteryl ester and triglyceride; their polar surface layers are made up of **apolipoproteins**, phospholipids and free cholesterol. They are classified according to their densities into four main types: the largest and least dense, **chylomicrons**, consist almost entirely of triglyceride; **very-low-density lipoproteins** (VLDL) consist largely of triglyceride; **low-density lipoproteins** (LDL) are cholesterol-rich; **high-density lipoproteins** (HDL) contain more cholesterol than triglyceride but apolipoproteins account for nearly half of their composition.

Lp(a) is an LDL-like lipoprotein in which an additional apolipoprotein, apo(a), is covalently linked to apoB. Apo(a) has close homology to plasminogen, and may compete with plasminogen for binding to fibrin. A resulting inhibition of thrombolysis could account for the role of Lp(a) as a risk factor for coronary artery disease.

APOLIPOPROTEINS

Apolipoproteins have several functions, including the binding and solubilization of lipids and the activation of enzymes: for example, chylomicrons contain apolipoprotein (apo) C-II, which activates **lipoprotein lipase** in the capillaries, and apoA-I on HDL activates **lecithin-cholesterol acyltransferase** (LCAT). They are also recognized by receptors on the surface of cells that utilize lipids: receptors in the liver recognize apoB-100 on LDL and apoB-48 on chylomicrons. The apolipoproteins are divided into five classes

Apolipoprotein content* of lipoproteins in fasting plasma				
	Chylomicrons	VLDL	LDL	HDL
ApoA-I	Tr	Tr	Tr	66
ApoA-II	Tr	Tr	Tr	20
ApoB	5–20	37	97	–
ApoC-I	15	3	Tr	3
ApoC-II	15	7	Tr	Tr
ApoC-III	40–50	40	2	4
ApoD	–	–	–	5
ApoE	4	13	1	1

*Per cent of total protein; Tr, trace.

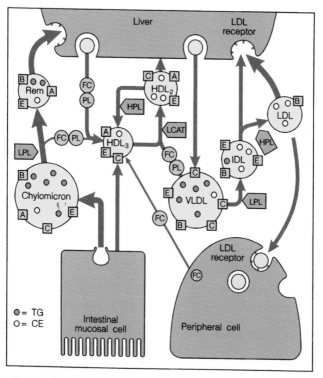

Tissue sites of origin and degradation and the intravascular metabolism of the lipoproteins. Rem, chylomicron remnant; LPL, lipoprotein lipase; HPL, hepatic lipase; FC, free cholesterol; PL, phospholipid; TG, triglyceride; CE, cholesteryl ester; A, B, C, E, apolipoproteins.

(A, B, C, D, and E), some of which are further divided. The presence of individual apolipoproteins on particular lipoproteins is related to the functions of that class of lipoprotein.

EXOGENOUS LIPID TRANSPORT

Exogenous or dietary fat (mainly triglyceride and cholesterol) is absorbed in the small intestine and incorporated in chylomicrons that enter the blood via the lymphatic pathway. Lipoprotein lipase, an enzyme found on the surface of endothelial cells in capillary beds serving muscle and adipose tissue, hydrolyzes the triglyceride in the chylomicrons; the **free fatty acid** released is taken up for oxidation or storage. Free cholesterol and phospholipids, surface components of the chylomicron released during hydrolysis, are incorporated into **HDL$_3$**. LCAT, a plasma enzyme, esterifies the cholesterol in HDL$_3$ in the conversion of this particle to HDL$_2$. HDL$_2$ then transfers the cholesterol back to the liver (see below). Cholesterol-rich **chylomicron remnants** are taken up by a receptor on the liver that binds the apoE on their surface.

Although dietary cholesterol does not contribute directly to high plasma cholesterol levels, it is possible that excessive cholesterol and saturated fat in the diet might lead to reduced production of LDL receptors by the liver and thus reduced uptake of the cholesterol-carrying LDL.

ENDOGENOUS LIPID TRANSPORT

Endogenously synthesized triglyceride and cholesterol are derived mainly from the liver and are transported to extrahepatic sites by VLDL. VLDL, like chylomicrons, are hydrolyzed by lipoprotein lipase; the resultant VLDL remnants are also called **intermediate-density lipoproteins** (IDL). Some of the IDL are removed from the circulation by the **B/E** or **LDL receptor**, which recognizes both the apoE and the apoB$_{100}$ on their surfaces. The remainder are further hydrolyzed by **hepatic lipase**, which converts them to LDL, the major cholesterol carrier in plasma. Some LDL is taken up by extrahepatic cells that require cholesterol but the majority is removed by LDL receptors in the liver.

Hepatic uptake of LDL not only determines the level of LDL in plasma but also controls the rate of synthesis of cholesterol by down-regulating the activity of **HMG CoA reductase** (β-hydroxy-β-methylglutaryl coenzyme A reductase). This enzyme catalyzes the conversion of HMG CoA to mevalonic acid, an early rate-limiting step on the cholesterol synthesis pathway. HMG CoA reductase activity is regulated by a negative feedback mechanism; it appears to be inversely related to cellular levels of oxysterol, an oxygenated cholesterol derivative. LDL-derived cholesterol also down-regulates the gene controlling the synthesis of LDL receptors. In turn, this causes a decrease in LDL uptake.

REVERSE TRANSPORT OF CHOLESTEROL

Reverse transport of cholesterol is mediated by HDL_3, which takes up excess free cholesterol from peripheral cells and is then converted by LCAT to larger HDL_2 (see above). Much of the resultant cholesteryl ester is then transferred to VLDL and LDL by the **cholesteryl ester transfer protein** (CETP) for eventual removal from plasma via the LDL receptor. The remainder is taken up directly by the liver, which requires a continuous supply for conversion into bile acids.

SUMMARY

The net result of these various metabolic steps is the transport of triglyceride to sites that require free fatty acids for provision of energy and the recycling of cholesterol between its sites of synthesis, utilization, and disposal. Genetic or environmental influences that accentuate input or retard disposal of the lipids inevitably lead to their accumulation in plasma. In some instances, defective clearance reflects mutations in genes encoding lipoprotein receptors or enzymes; in others the abnormality resides in apolipoproteins that normally act as ligands for receptors or cofactors for enzymes.

4 Epidemiology

GEOGRAPHIC PREVALENCE

Population studies have revealed high concentrations of total and LDL cholesterol in societies such as the USA and Finland, where diets are relatively high in saturated fat, and lower concentrations in societies such as China and Japan, where diets are relatively low in fat. LDL cholesterol concentrations rise significantly in Japanese who move to the USA, suggesting that diet and lifestyle may be more important factors than ethnic origin. In Finland, however, the high LDL concentrations may reflect a combination of dietary habits and an inherited susceptibility to increased uptake of dietary cholesterol. Moreover, hypercholesterolemia is more common in certain ethnic groups such as French-Canadians and Afrikaners, which is attributable to a gene founder effect with limited dilution of the gene in the general population of Quebec and South Africa.

HEREDITY

A number of specific genetic disorders affect lipoprotein levels. These are classified and discussed in Section 5 (*Primary hyperlipidemia*). Most of these hereditary disorders are inherited as autosomal dominant traits, and some are strongly associated with premature atherosclerosis.

▶ *A family tree should be constructed for each patient identified as having hyperlipidemia, and, when appropriate, other family members should be screened.*

SEX

After puberty, HDL-cholesterol levels are lower in men than in women, but triglyceride and LDL- and VLDL-cholesterol levels are higher. These differences are hormonally mediated: estrogens tend to lower LDL and raise HDL, whereas androgens have the opposite effect.

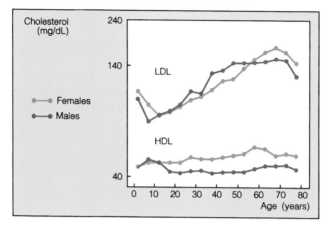

Mean LDL and HDL levels in men and women.

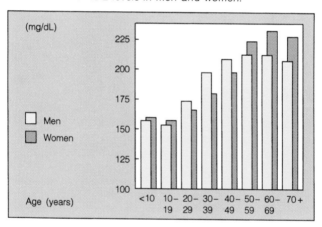

Plasma cholesterol concentrations in American white men and women according to age.

AGE

Plasma cholesterol concentrations rise rapidly during the first 6 months of life and then remain stable throughout childhood. LDL concentrations rise after puberty, reaching their peak in men between 50 and 60 and in women between 60 and 70 years of age.

5 Primary hyperlipidemia

PRIMARY HYPERCHOLESTEROLEMIAS

Familial hypercholesterolemia

Familial hypercholesterolemia results from inherited defects in the gene encoding the LDL receptor, leading to defective clearance of cholesterol-carrying LDL from the circulation [5].

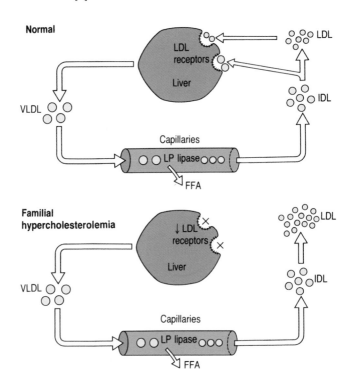

LP lipase, lipoprotein lipase; FFA, free fatty acids.

People with **heterozygous familial hypercholesterolemia** have 50% fewer high-affinity LDL receptors on hepatic and peripheral cells. This condition occurs in one out of 500 people in Western Europe and North America. It is an autosomal dominant trait with complete phenotypic expression in childhood. Sufferers often have LDL-cholesterol levels that are two to three times above the normal range, with a total cholesterol concentration of 300 to 500 mg/dL.

Very rarely, the inheritance of two mutant genes causes **homozygous familial hypercholesterolemia**, which is usually detected before the patient is 10 years old by the presence of tuberous and tendon xanthomas. Plasma total cholesterol levels reach >600 to 800 mg/dL and there is a primary increase in LDL cholesterol. Without treatment, coronary atherosclerosis develops by 10 to 15 years of age and myocardial infarction has been reported as early as $1\frac{1}{2}$ to 3 years.

A few patients have abnormalities in the protein component of LDL, resulting in impaired binding of apolipoprotein B to the LDL receptor. This condition, known as **familial defective apolipoprotein B100**, also causes primary hypercholesterolemia. The population frequency of this disorder is unknown but may be as common as one in 600.

▶ *It is strongly recommended that patients with familial hypercholesterolemia be referred to a lipid clinic for optimal counseling and management.*

Polygenic hypercholesterolemia is a term applied to patients with evidence of primary hypercholesterolemia but no bimodality in cholesterol concentrations in their family, suggesting a multiple-gene etiology. They are at increased risk of atherosclerosis because of elevated total- and LDL-cholesterol levels.

Familial hyperalphalipoproteinemia is an autosomal dominantly inherited trait leading to raised HDL cholesterol levels, generally ≥75 mg/dL. It appears to confer longevity and low CHD risk. No treatment is required.

Cholesterol ester hydrolase deficiency, an autosomal recessive disorder, results in hypercholesterolemia and concurrent hepatosplenomegaly. **Betasitosterolemia**, in which absorption of dietary sterols is abnormally increased, causes tendon xanthomas and modest hyper-cholesterolemia.

PRIMARY MIXED (COMBINED) HYPERLIPIDEMIAS

Familial combined hyperlipidemia is inherited as an auto-somal dominant trait but shows incomplete expression in childhood. It appears to be due to an inherent overproduc-tion of VLDL by the liver that may lead to elevated levels of LDL cholesterol. Patients may show raised LDL, raised VLDL, or both. It is associated with increased CHD risk, per-haps 10 years later than that seen in heterozygous familial hypercholesterolemia. The gene frequency is estimated at 1% in Western Europe and North America.

Combined hyperlipidemia with raised VLDL and LDL can also occur in **hyperapobetalipoproteinemia**.

Type III hyperlipoproteinemia, also known as **familial dys-betalipoproteinemia**, is relatively uncommon and is char-acterized by abnormal cholesterol-rich VLDL and chylo-micron remnant particles in plasma. This disorder predis-poses the patient to premature atherosclerosis. Cholesterol levels of 250 to 770 mg/dL and triglyceride levels of 530 to 1770 mg/dL are common. Most patients are homozygous for apolipoprotein EII, which results in impaired binding of EII-containing particles to hepatic LDL and apolipoprotein E receptors. Patients may have a coexisting disorder — such as obesity, diabetes, hypothyroidism, and excess al-cohol consumption — that increases hepatic VLDL syn-thesis. They may also have a second hereditary disorder — such as familial combined hyperlipidemia — that in-creases hepatic VLDL production. The clinical frequency is 1 : 5000 to 1 :10,000. It is extremely rare in childhood and premenopausal women, and estrogen replacement therapy may provide some protection for postmenopausal women.

PRIMARY HYPERTRIGLYCERIDEMIAS

Familial hypertriglyceridemia is inherited as an autosomal dominant trait with incomplete expression in childhood. Patients have either increased triglycerides due to raised VLDL levels (phenotype IV) or more severe increases in triglycerides and cholesterol due to accumulation of both

VLDL and chylomicrons (phenotype V). LDL and HDL concentrations are often low; VLDL triglyceride synthesis in the liver appears to be increased. Unlike familial combined hyperlipidemia, familial hypertriglyceridemia may not produce an increased risk of premature atherosclerosis. It can be exacerbated by excessive alcohol consumption, increasing body weight, or certain drugs, leading to increased levels of chylomicrons and a phenotypic type V pattern. It is common among European and American adults, in whom coexistent problems often exacerbate familial hypertriglyceridemia.

Familial lipoprotein lipase deficiency, also known as **familial type I hyperlipoproteinemia**, is rare. Inherited as an autosomal recessive disorder, it is usually detected in childhood because of bouts of abdominal pain and hepatosplenomegaly and is characterized by markedly elevated triglycerides with chylomicronemia. Heterozygotic patients have a 50% decrease in enzyme activity, leading to mild hypertriglyceridemia or a pattern similar to that seen in familial combined hyperlipidemia. Frequency is estimated at one in a million.

The inherited lack of apolipoprotein CII, a disorder known as **familial apolipoprotein CII deficiency**, may also cause severe hypertriglyceridemia, with a type I or V phenotype.

DISORDERS OF HIGH-DENSITY LIPOPROTEINS

Familial hypoalphalipoproteinemia is relatively common, with a population frequency of 1:400 to 500. It is characterized by plasma HDL levels of <20 to 30 mg/dL, but normal or only slightly raised triglyceride levels. This disorder is associated with an increased risk of premature CHD.

A number of rarer familial syndromes also exist in which levels of HDL and its constituent apolipoproteins are severely reduced. These include **LCAT deficiency**, **familial apolipoprotein AI-CIII deficiency**, **Tangier disease**, **HDL deficiency with planar xanthomas**, **fish-eye disease** and **apolipoprotein AI$_{milano}$**.

The patient with significantly reduced HDL levels should be referred to a lipid specialist for evaluation.

6 Causes of secondary hyperlipidemia

Hyperlipidemia can be attributed to a number of causes such as diet, hormonal disturbances, drugs, or coexisting diseases. However, in many patients these factors merely exacerbate an underlying genetic abnormality.

DIET

Saturated fats raise plasma concentrations of LDL cholesterol and potentiate the hypercholesterolemic effects of dietary cholesterol [6]. Foods high in saturated fats include milk and dairy products, animal fats and organ meats. Diets high in **carbohydrates** and low in saturated fats are associated with low LDL cholesterol levels, but these diets also tend to raise plasma triglycerides and lower HDL cholesterol levels. (See Section 14, *Dietary management*.)

A modest **alcohol** intake raises HDL cholesterol but may also raise plasma triglycerides.

Effects of diet on plasma lipids				
Dietary component	**Cholesterol**			**Triglycerides**
	Total	**LDL**	**HDL**	
Saturated fatty acids (C14, C16)	↑	↑	± ↑	—
Monounsaturated fatty acids	↓	↓	—	—
Polyunsaturated (ω6) fatty acids	↓	↓	± ↓	—
Polyunsaturated (ω3) fatty acids	± ↓	± ↑ or ↓	± ↓	↓
Cholesterol	↑	↑	± ↑	—
Soluble fiber	↓	↓	—	—
Complex carbohydrate	↓	↓	± ↓	± ↑
Alcohol	↑	—	± ↑	± ↑
Excess calories	↑	± ↑	± ↓	↑

↑, increased; ↓, decreased; ± ↑, slightly increased; ± ↓, slightly decreased.

Consumption of large amounts of boiled **coffee** may have a hypercholesterolemic effect; a similar effect is not seen with tea.

TOBACCO

Habitual smoking is associated with a 4 to 12 mg/dL decrease in plasma HDL concentrations and a tendency for triglycerides to rise slightly.

▶ *Patients should be advised to stop smoking because of the high CHD risk as well as a high risk for cancer and lung disease.*

WEIGHT

An excessive intake of calories leads to increased plasma concentrations of triglycerides and reduced HDL cholesterol. (See Section 14, *Dietary management*.)

PREGNANCY

Cholesterol (LDL and VLDL) and triglyceride concentrations increase in the second and third trimesters of pregnancy and return to normal *post partum*. In women with primary hyperlipidemia, increases can be severe.

OTHER DISEASES

Hypothyroidism

Hypothyroidism is an important cause of secondary hypercholesterolemia and can also lead to combined hyperlipidemia or, less commonly, severe hypertriglyceridemia. Its treatment usually leads to normalization of plasma lipid levels.

Diabetes mellitus

Patients with poorly controlled diabetes mellitus may present with severe hypertriglyceridemia. Insulin is necessary for the production of lipoprotein lipase, and its deficiency also leads to increased lipolysis in adipose tissue with a resulting flux of fatty acids to the liver. This reaction can be reversed by hydration and insulin administration. Mild hypertriglyceridemia is also seen in patients with non–insulin-dependent diabetes mellitus. In these patients, hyperinsulinism is associated with increased hepatic VLDL production.

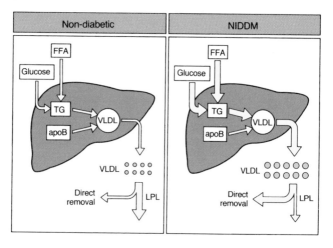

NIDDM, non–insulin-dependent diabetes mellitus; TG, triglyceride; FFA, free fatty acids; LPL, lipoprotein lipase.

Hypoalbuminemia

Hypoalbuminemia due to renal loss (**nephrotic syndrome**) or loss from the gastrointestinal tract (**protein-losing enteropathy**) promotes an increase in the production of VLDL and LDL and can lead to combined hyperlipidemia or hypercholesterolemia.

▶ *The risk of CHD is increased in patients with nephrotic syndrome, and chronic nephrotic syndrome often justifies treatment with lipid-lowering drugs.*

Chronic renal failure

Uremia is often associated with raised cholesterol and triglyceride levels, partly because of an acquired defect of lipoprotein lipase. Chronic hyperlipidemia after renal transplantation is common and can be attributed in part to the hyperlipidemic effects of prednisone and cyclosporine.

Obstructive liver disease

Cholestasis may be associated with severe hypercholesterolemia in which an abnormal lipoprotein (lipoprotein X) accumulates in plasma. Impaired biliary excretion of cholesterol and bile acids is the cause.

▶ *With cholestasis, drug therapy is often ineffective. A consultation with a lipid specialist should be sought for such patients. The patients may benefit from plasmapheresis.*

Drugs

Plasma lipid and lipoprotein concentrations can be influenced by a number of prescription medications.

Effects of drugs on lipid and lipoprotein concentrations				
Drug	**Total chol**	**TG**	**LDL chol**	**HDL chol**
Corticosteroids	↑	↑↑	± ↑	± ↑
Estrogens	↑	↑	↓	↑
Progestins	± ↑	± ↑	± ↑	↓
Androgens	↓	±	↑	↓
Beta blockers (without ISA)	↑	↑	± ↑	↓
Thiazide diuretics	↑	↑	± ↑	↓
Vitamin A derivatives	± ↑	↑↑	↓	↓
Cyclosporine	↑	—	↑	—
Phenytoin	↑	—	—	↑
Barbiturates	↑	—	—	↑

Chol, cholesterol; TG, triglyceride; ISA, intrinsic sympathomimetic activity; ↑, increased; ↓, decreased; ± ↑, slightly increased; ± ↓, slightly decreased; ↑↑, greatly increased; —, no change.

7 Lipids and cardiovascular risk

LIPIDS AND RISK

Atherosclerosis leading to CHD is currently the most common cause of death in America and Western Europe. Its incidence correlates with both abnormal lipid levels and raised blood pressure. People with total serum cholesterol levels of less than 150 mg/dL are rarely affected.

The **Multiple Risk Factor Intervention Trial (MRFIT)** has shown that the risk of CHD is more or less continuous over the whole range of serum cholesterol levels:

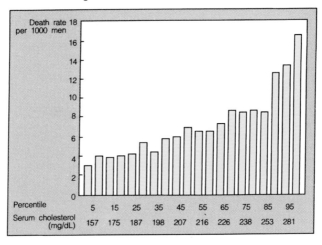

This graph shows that CHD risk rises appreciably when serum cholesterol exceeds 250 mg/dL and even more steeply when it rises above 280 mg/dL. After 10½ years of the trial, cardiovascular mortality was reduced by 10.6% and mortality from all causes by 7.7% in the 'special intervention' group (which received advice on reduction of risk factors) when compared with the 'usual care' group.

The **Seven Countries Study** [7] showed correlations between the incidence of CHD in men between 40 and 59 years and the proportion whose total serum cholesterol level exceeded 250 mg/dL (see graph on facing page). It was suggested that differences in the percentage of a population with high cholesterol levels (ranging from

7% in Japan to 56% in Finland) were largely due to differences in the ratio of saturated to unsaturated fats in the diet.

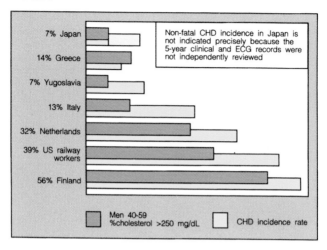

Non-fatal CHD incidence in Japan is not indicated precisely because the 5-year clinical and ECG records were not independently reviewed

| ■ | Men 40-59 %cholesterol >250 mg/dL | □ | CHD incidence rate |

The **Framingham Study** [8] showed that the risk of CHD was markedly increased in people who had hypercholesterolemia, hypertension or hyperglycemia, or who smoked cigarettes. It also showed a strong inverse correlation between HDL cholesterol and CHD in both men and women:

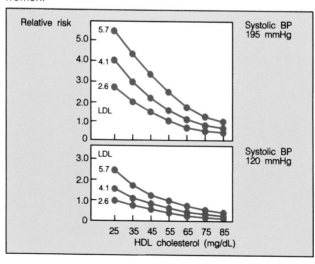

LIPIDS AND ATHEROSCLEROSIS

As well as showing a relationship between lipid levels and CHD, studies show that treatment of hyperlipidemia can reduce or reverse lipid-induced atherosclerosis. This section illustrates the effect of lipids on the development of atherosclerosis and summarizes evidence that lipid-lowering therapy can induce regression of atherosclerosis.

The pathogenesis of atherosclerosis

The characteristic lesion of atherosclerosis is the fatty fibrous plaque. The causal role of LDL in atherogenesis is illustrated below:

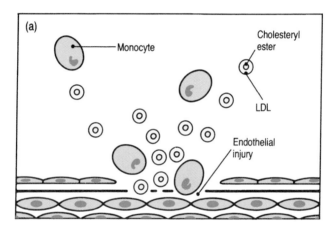

(a) LDL accumulates at the site of endothelial injury, which attracts blood monocytes to the site. (b) The monocytes penetrate the intima to become macrophages and ingest the LDL together with its accompanying cholesteryl esters, giving rise to foam cells. (c) Platelets adhere and release growth factors. (d) Smooth-muscle cells migrate from the media and secrete collagen, forming a fibrous plaque. Eventual necrosis of foam cells results in hydrolysis of cholesteryl esters and the formation of cholesteryl ester crystals within the core of the mature plaque.

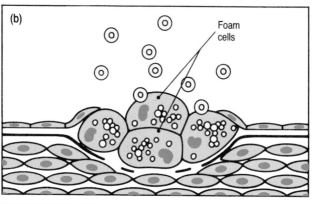

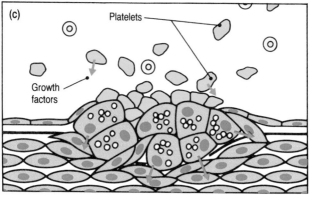

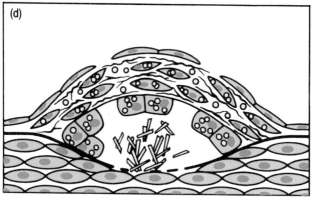

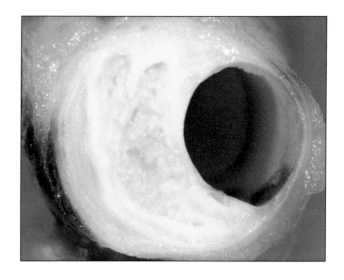

The fatty fibrous plaque.

Fatal cases may be caused by hemorrhage into or on the luminal surface or fracture, leading to thrombosis. When symptoms of coronary insufficiency occur, the lumen of at least one branch of a coronary artery is usually narrowed to less than 25% of its original diameter by such plaques. Fibrous tissue is the main component, but up to 45% of the lesion consists of lipid, mainly cholesterol, derived almost entirely from the blood.

REGRESSION OF ATHEROSCLEROSIS

Until recently, angiographic evidence that regression of human atherosclerosis could be achieved was not available. However, it is now apparent that effective lipid-lowering therapy can influence both the progression and the regression of atherosclerotic lesions.

In the National Heart, Lung, and Blood Institute (NHLBI) **Type II Coronary Intervention Trial** [9], a moderate decrease in LDL cholesterol and a modest increase in the HDL:LDL ratio by cholestyramine treatment over a 5-year period dramatically curtailed the progression of coronary lesions. In the **Cholesterol Lowering Atherosclerosis Study (CLAS)** [10], a larger decrease in LDL and increase in the HDL:LDL ratio by a combination of colestipol and nicotinic acid over 2–3 years actually caused a significant lesion regression. Most recently, the **Familial Atherosclerosis Treatment Study (FATS)** [11] demonstrated that, compared with those receiving conventional treatment, high-risk patients treated with a combination of lovastatin and colestipol, or niacin and colestipol, experienced a dramatic decrease in lesion progression and an increase in atherosclerotic regression.

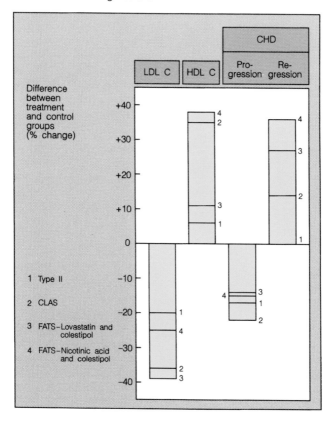

EFFECTS OF TREATMENT ON MORBIDITY AND MORTALITY

Several studies have demonstrated that treating abnormal lipid levels will reduce cardiovascular morbidity and mortality.

In the **Lipid Research Clinics Coronary Primary Prevention Trial (LRC-CPPT)** [12] more than 3800 asymptomatic, hypercholesterolemic middle-aged men were placed on low-fat diets and then randomized to treatment with either placebo or cholestyramine. Over the 7-year trial, the cholestyramine group reduced its mean total and LDL-cholesterol levels by 9 and 12%, respectively, when compared with the placebo group. Furthermore, the cholestyramine group had 19% fewer CHD events than the placebo group. These findings indicated a 1:2 ratio between the degree of total-cholesterol lowering and CHD reduction.

The 4081 subjects in the 5-year **Helsinki Heart Study** [13], a double-blind, randomized trial, were also asymptomatic, middle-aged men with hypercholesterolemia. Treatment with gemfibrozil lowered total cholesterol levels by 10%, LDL by 11% and triglycerides by 35%, and increased HDL levels by 11% when compared with treatment with placebo. On the basis of the results obtained in the LRC-CPPT, the gemfibrozil-treated group would have been expected to experience 20% fewer CHD events than the placebo group. However, 34% fewer cardiac deaths and non-fatal myocardial infarctions were observed. It was determined that raising HDL-cholesterol levels had an effect on reducing the incidence of CHD that was independent of and additive to that of lowering total and LDL-cholesterol levels.

Recent reports from three clinical studies strongly suggest that cholesterol lowering will reduce total mortality.

As part of the NHLBI's **Coronary Drug Project** [14], 1119 male survivors of myocardial infarction were treated with niacin and 2789 male survivors with placebo. At the end of the 6-year trial, the total cholesterol levels of the niacin group were 10% lower than those of the placebo group. In a 15-year follow-up, almost 9 years after the trial's completion, total mortality in the niacin group was 11% lower than that in the placebo group. This difference was linked to the earlier cholesterol-lowering effect of the drug.

In the **Oslo Study Diet and Antismoking Trial** [15], more than 1200 middle-aged, hypercholesterolemic men were randomized to an intervention or a control group. After 5 years, total cholesterol levels in the intervention group were down by an average of 13% compared with 3% in the control group. Also, the rate of coronary events was 47% lower in the intervention group. A follow-up some 3 to 4 years after the completion of the trial showed that these trends had continued: the intervention group experienced 45% fewer coronary events than did the placebo group, and the difference between the two groups' total mortality rates had widened.

In the 5-year **Stockholm Ischemic Heart Study** [16], more than 560 myocardial infarction survivors, half of whom had hypertriglyceridemia, were randomized to a control group or a group treated with clofibrate and niacin. The treatment group experienced 26% fewer deaths than did the control group, with 36% fewer deaths due to ischemic heart disease.

8 Other risk factors for coronary heart disease

A number of risk factors in addition to hyperlipidemia are associated with CHD, hypertension and smoking being the most clearly established. CHD risk also increases with age, has a strong genetic component, and is greater in men than women until menopause. Sedentary habits, obesity, and diabetes mellitus are also important.

▶ *In patients with hypercholesterolemia, special attention should be paid to the management of other CHD risk factors, such as hypertension, smoking, diabetes, low HDL levels, and obesity. Attention should also be paid to age, sex, and family history of premature CHD.*

HYPERTENSION AND SMOKING

Hypertension is a strong independent risk factor for the development of atherosclerosis and CHD. The presence of hypertension more than doubles the CHD risk at any given level of serum cholesterol, and a similar, but smaller, increment is attributable to cigarette smoking. The coexistence of hypertension and cigarette smoking with hypercholesterolemia results in a multiplicative, rather than an additive, increase in risk, as illustrated below:

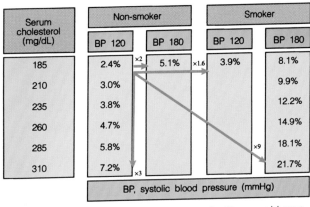

Serum cholesterol (mg/dL)	Non-smoker		Smoker	
	BP 120	BP 180	BP 120	BP 180
185	2.4%	5.1%	3.9%	8.1%
210	3.0%			9.9%
235	3.8%			12.2%
260	4.7%			14.9%
285	5.8%			18.1%
310	7.2%			21.7%

BP, systolic blood pressure (mmHg)

Probability of developing CHD in 8 years in 45-year-old men with normal ECG in the Framingham study according to serum cholesterol, blood pressure, and smoking habits.

The relative risk of CHD in hypercholesterolemic, hypertensive smokers is nine times that in their normocholesterolemic, normotensive, non-smoking counterparts.

HYPERGLYCEMIA AND DIABETES

An association between diabetes and CHD has been established in western societies. Severe hypertriglyceridemia, rapidly responsive to insulin, can occur often in juvenile-onset diabetes. Hypertriglyceridemia and a reduced level of HDL cholesterol are common in adult-onset diabetics, and these factors probably contribute to the increased risk of CHD. Impaired glucose tolerance often accompanies type IV or V hyperlipidemia, implying insulin resistance.

AGE AND SEX

The *absolute risk* of CHD increases with age and is much greater at age 55 than age 20. However, serum cholesterol elevations cause a steeper increase in the *relative risk* of CHD for 20-year-olds than they do for 55-year-olds. Thus, the benefits of therapeutic intervention will probably be greater if intervention is started sooner rather than later in life.

At any given level of serum cholesterol, the risk of CHD in men is about three times that in women of the same age until menopause. About 5 to 10 years after menopause, the risks become comparable in both sexes. This relatively lower risk in premenopausal women should be remembered when considering intervention.

FAMILY HISTORY

A family history of premature CHD (before 55 years of age) is an important risk factor. In many instances this is a result of an inherited tendency toward hyperlipidemia due to increased LDL, VLDL, or triglyceride production, or a decrease in LDL receptor activity, or toward a decreased level of HDL. Increased levels of Lp(a), an LDL-like lipoprotein with thrombogenic properties, may also be a factor.

9 Screening

Most people with elevated lipid levels are asymptomatic. Therefore, screening is essential to identify those who can be treated to reduce their lipid levels and thus their risk of cardiovascular morbidity and mortality.

Those identified from public screening as having raised lipid levels should be referred to a physician.

Opportunistic screening of all patients over age 20 should be carried out as part of routine medical care along the guidelines set by the NCEP (see facing page). Total cholesterol levels should be measured when the patient first sees his or her clinician. However, treatment should not be based on measurements taken during illness or periods of weight loss, both of which alter values, or during pregnancy, when lipid levels are elevated.

If opportunistic screening is impractical, **selective screening** of high-risk individuals should be undertaken. Selective screening should identify those with familial hypercholesterolemia.

Selective screening for hyperlipidemia
First-degree relatives of patients with hyperlipidemia
Presence of xanthomas or xanthelasma in patient or first-degree relative
Family history of coronary artery disease before age 50 (men) or 60 (women)
Corneal arcus before age 50

Measurements should also be taken in patients with atherosclerosis or with other disorders that increase the risk of its development, such as hypertension and diabetes.

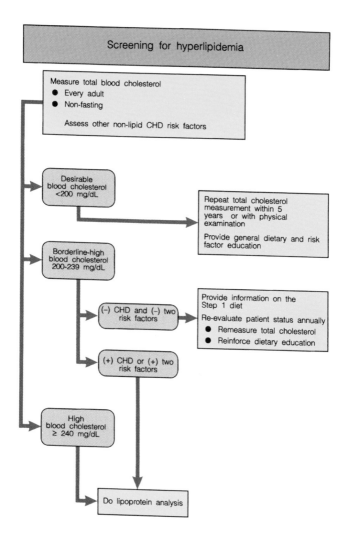

10 Measurement of blood lipids and lipoproteins

Important: Raised levels should always be confirmed by repeated lipoprotein analyses, 1 to 8 weeks apart, before treatment is begun.

CHOLESTEROL MEASUREMENT

There are two approaches to measuring total cholesterol:

1 *Desk-top analyzer (finger-stick)*, which uses finger-pricked blood. For results to be reliable, the machine must be in regular use and be included in a quality-control program. This method is convenient because the measurement can be taken in a clinician's office or at a temporary screening site such as a school, church, shopping mall, or work place. In most cases, total cholesterol can be measured within 5 minutes.
2 *Laboratory lipoprotein analysis (venipuncture)*. This analysis ideally requires a 12-hour fast and should be carried out by a reputable hospital or clinic laboratory [17].

▶ *Determining the full lipid profile is more expensive than measuring total cholesterol alone, and so the desk-top analyzer is useful for initial screening. However, a lipoprotein analysis is needed to determine the appropriate treatment based on the NCEP management guidelines.*

LIPOPROTEIN ANALYSIS

Lipids can be analyzed in serum or plasma, preferably with minimal venostasis. Since a lipid profile includes measurement of triglycerides, a 12-hour fast is required before the screening.

If the sample is translucent, the triglyceride level is probably normal, but the cholesterol level may be normal or raised. Hypertriglyceridemic samples are usually hazy or opaque.

Chylomicrons form a surface film on standing, whereas VLDLs remain diffuse.

HDL-cholesterol levels should also be measured after first precipitating and centrifuging down the VLDL and LDL. Values for LDL cholesterol can be derived from HDL cholesterol and triglyceride levels rather than measured directly, according to the calculation on page 38.

Cholesterol and triglycerides are usually measured enzymatically in large autoanalyzers. Current recommendations are that inaccuracy should not exceed ±3 to 5% and the coefficient of variation should be less than 5%. Most desk-top analyzers, when used properly, meet these requirements.

Day-to-day variations in an individual's levels range from 4 to 12% for total and HDL cholesterol and from 13 to 14% for triglyceride. There is both biological variability (see table below) and analytic variability, depending on the method employed. Serum lipids tend to be higher in winter than in summer. Other factors that influence serum lipids are listed below.

Physiological and environmental influences on serum lipids				
	Total C	**LDL C**	**HDL C**	**TG**
Aging	↑	↑		↑
Female sex			↑	↓
Obesity	↑		↓	↑
Exercise		↓	↑	↓
Trauma	↓	↓		↑
Saturated fat	↑	↑		
Monounsaturated fat	↓	↓		
Polyunsaturated fat:				
ω6	↓	↓	↓	
ω3	↑	↑		↓
Alcohol			↑	↑
C, cholesterol; TG, triglyceride; ↑, increased; ↓, decreased.				

11 Physical signs

In a minority of patients with primary hyperlipidemia, physical signs can suggest a diagnosis, which should be confirmed by a lipoprotein analysis.

PRIMARY HYPERCHOLESTEROLEMIA

There usually are no physical abnormalities in **familial hypercholesterolemia** during childhood except in homozygotes, in whom planar xanthomas in digital webs or behind the knees are common.

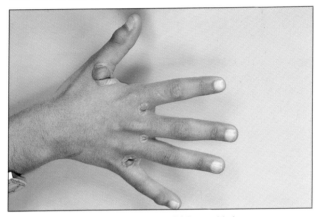

Planar xanthomas in a 12-year-old boy with homozygous familial hypercholesterolemia.

Recurring Achilles tendinitis, usually exercise-related, occurs in roughly 50% of patients with heterozygous familial hypercholesterolemia, frequently first in the late teens or early 20s. The typical tendon xanthomas become more prominent with age, often involving extensor tendons of the hands, Achilles tendons, or, less commonly, the patellar tendons and olecranon.

Xanthelasma occurs in 20% of these patients, but is not specific for familial hypercholesterolemia. Corneal arcus in caucasian patients under 35 years of age is diagnostic, but not always present.

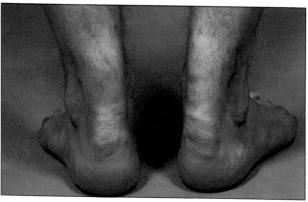

Achilles tendon xanthomas in a 47-year-old man with heterozygous familial hypercholesterolemia.

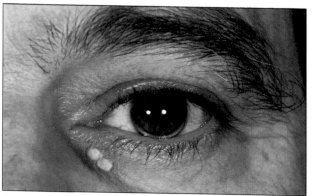

Corneal arcus and xanthelasma in the same 47-year-old man.

Patients reported to date with **familial defective apolipoprotein B100** have had modest primary hypercholesterolemia. A few of these patients had tendon xanthomas.

PRIMARY MIXED (COMBINED) HYPERLIPIDEMIA
There are no characteristic physical findings in **familial combined hyperlipidemia** that can alert the clinician to this disorder.

Type III hyperlipoproteinemia is associated with very characteristic xanthomas, although not in all patients. The most common skin manifestations are a yellow-orange discoloration in the palmar creases of the hands.

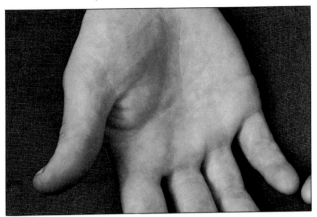

Yellowish palmar striae in a 35-year-old man with type III hyperlipoproteinemia.

Tuberoeruptive xanthomas (see facing page), which consist of raised 0.5-cm nodular lesions in areas of pressure, particularly the knees and elbows, are very characteristic. As these lesions become larger, they coalesce into tuberous xanthomas.

PRIMARY HYPERTRIGLYCERIDEMIA

Many patients with severe **familial hypertriglyceridemia** (triglycerides > 1750 mg/dL) are asymptomatic, but abdominal pain or tenderness of the liver and spleen are common, and hepatomegaly is sometimes noted on physical examination. In patients with triglyceride concentrations > 1325 mg/dL, lipemia retinalis, a pinkish-white discoloration of the retinal vessels, is seen on fundoscopic examination, while eruptive xanthomas, small yellow-white papules on an erythematous base, may be seen on the arms, buttocks, and thighs.

Characteristic manifestations of **familial lipoprotein lipase deficiency** in early childhood may include eruptive xan-

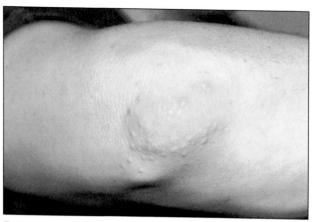

Tuberoeruptive xanthomas in the same patient.

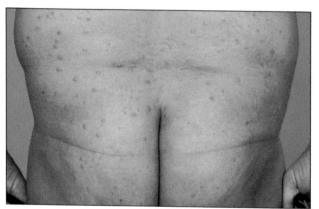

Eruptive xanthomas in a 33-year-old man with type V hyperlipoproteinemia.

thomas in response to breast-feeding, abdominal pain, pancreatitis, and hepatosplenomegaly. Diagnosis is based on family history and the documentation of reduced or virtually absent levels of lipoprotein lipase in post-heparin plasma or adipose tissue.

12 Supplementary investigations

Elevated total cholesterol levels should be confirmed with a lipoprotein analysis that measures total cholesterol, HDL, and triglycerides. LDL can then be calculated as follows:

$$LDL\ C\ =\ total\ C\ -\ HDL\ C\ -\ \frac{TG}{5}\ mg/dL$$

(C, cholesterol; TG, triglyceride. Note: this calculation cannot be done if TG > 400 mg/dL. The presence of chylomicrons in non-fasting samples will produce a spurious LDL level.)

Patients can usefully be grouped into three broad categories:

Category I
Increased total cholesterol and normal triglyceride levels

Category II
Increased total cholesterol and increased triglyceride levels

Category III
Increased total cholesterol and increased triglyceride levels, where the triglyceride concentrations are three to five times higher than the cholesterol and the plasma looks lipemic

For diagnostic purposes, the results obtained can be interpreted according to the three general flowcharts on the following pages. These outline the diagnostic course of action to be taken for each of the three broad categories.

Before the physician embarks on treatment (based on the NCEP and NIH Consensus guidelines; see pages 31 and 42), causes of secondary hyperlipidemia should be looked for and treated. In many cases, this will lead to normalization of lipid levels (see Section 6, *Causes of secondary hyperlipidemia*).

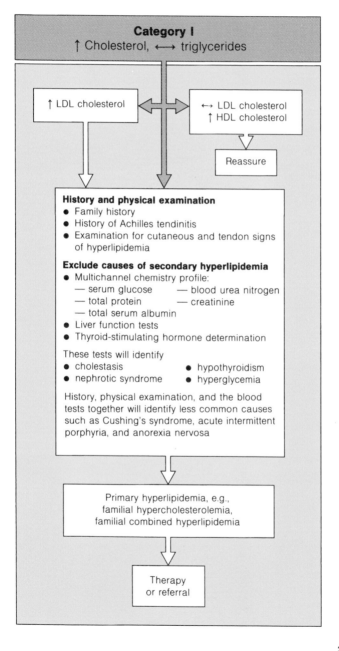

Category I
↑ Cholesterol, ←→ triglycerides

↑ LDL cholesterol

←→ LDL cholesterol
↑ HDL cholesterol

Reassure

History and physical examination
- Family history
- History of Achilles tendinitis
- Examination for cutaneous and tendon signs of hyperlipidemia

Exclude causes of secondary hyperlipidemia
- Multichannel chemistry profile:
  — serum glucose   — blood urea nitrogen
  — total protein   — creatinine
  — total serum albumin
- Liver function tests
- Thyroid-stimulating hormone determination

These tests will identify
- cholestasis   ● hypothyroidism
- nephrotic syndrome   ● hyperglycemia

History, physical examination, and the blood tests together will identify less common causes such as Cushing's syndrome, acute intermittent porphyria, and anorexia nervosa

Primary hyperlipidemia, e.g., familial hypercholesterolemia, familial combined hyperlipidemia

Therapy or referral

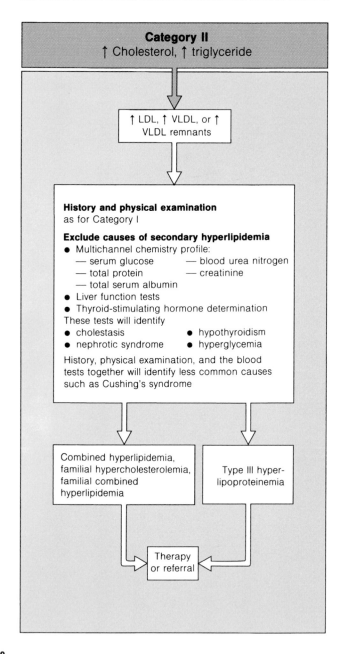

Category II
↑ Cholesterol, ↑ triglyceride

↑ LDL, ↑ VLDL, or ↑ VLDL remnants

History and physical examination
as for Category I

Exclude causes of secondary hyperlipidemia
● Multichannel chemistry profile:
 — serum glucose — blood urea nitrogen
 — total protein — creatinine
 — total serum albumin
● Liver function tests
● Thyroid-stimulating hormone determination
These tests will identify
● cholestasis ● hypothyroidism
● nephrotic syndrome ● hyperglycemia

History, physical examination, and the blood tests together will identify less common causes such as Cushing's syndrome

Combined hyperlipidemia, familial hypercholesterolemia, familial combined hyperlipidemia

Type III hyperlipoproteinemia

Therapy or referral

Category III
↑ Cholesterol, ↑↑ triglycerides >5 times normal, plasma lipemic

↑ VLDL
↑ chylomicrons

History and physical examination
- Family history
- History of abdominal pain
- History of pancreatitis
- Examination for cutaneous and tendon signs of hyperlipidemia

Exclude causes of secondary hyperlipidemia
- Multichannel chemistry profile and thyroid-stimulating hormone determination (as for Categories I and II)

- Also look for
  — poorly controlled diabetes
  — drug therapy (estrogens, thiazide diuretics, beta blockers, corticosteroids)
  — excess alcohol consumption

Type V hyperlipidemia
(familial hypertriglyceridemia, familial combined hyperlipidemia)

Therapy or referral

13 When to treat

Treatment of elevated cholesterol levels should be based on the algorithms on page 31 and below. These algorithms, designed by the NCEP, categorize a patient's risk of CHD on the basis of his or her total cholesterol and then LDL cholesterol levels.

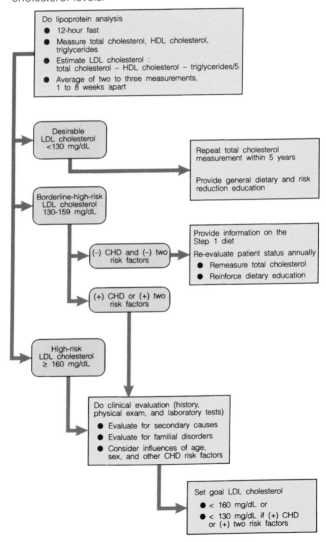

Do lipoprotein analysis
- 12-hour fast
- Measure total cholesterol, HDL cholesterol, triglycerides
- Estimate LDL cholesterol : total cholesterol – HDL cholesterol – triglycerides/5
- Average of two to three measurements, 1 to 8 weeks apart

Desirable
LDL cholesterol
<130 mg/dL

Repeat total cholesterol measurement within 5 years

Provide general dietary and risk reduction education

Borderline-high-risk
LDL cholesterol
130-159 mg/dL

(–) CHD and (–) two risk factors

Provide information on the Step 1 diet
Re-evaluate patient status annually
- Remeasure total cholesterol
- Reinforce dietary education

(+) CHD or (+) two risk factors

High-risk
LDL cholesterol
≥ 160 mg/dL

Do clinical evaluation (history, physical exam, and laboratory tests)
- Evaluate for secondary causes
- Evaluate for familial disorders
- Consider influences of age, sex, and other CHD risk factors

Set goal LDL cholesterol
- < 160 mg/dL or
- < 130 mg/dL if (+) CHD or (+) two risk factors

Factors for high-risk status for CHD

Definite CHD as indicated by:
- A previous heart attack
- Angina pectoris

Two other CHD risk factors:
- Family history of premature CHD (heart attack or sudden death before age 55 years in a parent, brother, or sister)
- Family history of stroke or vascular disease
- Male sex
- Hypertension
- Cigarette smoking (> 10 cigarettes per day)
- Diabetes mellitus
- Low HDL levels (< 35 mg/dL)
- Severe obesity (> 30% overweight)

For example, a patient with a total cholesterol level of less than 200 mg/dL is thought generally to have a low risk of CHD. In such a case, the patient should recheck his or her cholesterol levels within 5 years, or annually if possible, and learn some basic dietary steps that will help prevent the cholesterol level from rising.

In contrast, a patient with a total cholesterol level of over 240 mg/dL and an LDL level subsequently determined to be over 160 mg/dL is considered to have a high risk for CHD. This patient should have a thorough clinical evaluation, be placed on dietary therapy, and, if diet alone proves insufficient, on drug therapy as well.

THE GOALS OF TREATMENT
The **immediate goal of treatment** is to reduce elevated total and LDL cholesterol levels to desirable ranges.

The **long-term goal of treatment** and the rationale for intervention are to reduce the risk as well as the progression of atherosclerotic heart disease.

There are other clinical goals in the treatment of hyperlipidemia. Successful treatment of severe hypertriglyceridemia (phenotype V) reduces the risk of life-threatening pancreatitis. Treatment of phenotypes III and V reduces tuberous and eruptive xanthomas, respectively. Xanthelasmas and xanthomas that appear in phenotype II may also regress in response to lipid-lowering treatment.

14 Dietary management

Dietary advice is the first step in the treatment of all forms of hyperlipidemia and is often successful.

Patients with high-risk (>240 mg/dL) or borderline–high (200 to 239 mg/dL) cholesterol levels should be put on a lipid-lowering diet, such as the AHA's Step 1 and Step 2 diets. The Step 2 diet should be prescribed if the Step 1 diet is not effective after 3 months. This more stringent diet requires the assistance of a registered dietitian.

The aim of these diets is to reduce the consumption of fat, saturated fat, and cholesterol, while increasing the consumption of mono- or polyunsaturated fats and carbohydrates. Caloric intake should also be monitored to help maintain an ideal body weight.

Dietary components of Step 1 and Step 2 diets	
Step 1 diet	
Total fat	<30% of total calories
Saturated fatty acids	<10% of total calories
Polyunsaturated fatty acids	Up to 10% of total calories
Monounsaturated fatty acids	10–15% of total calories
Carbohydrates	50–60% of total calories
Protein	10–20% of total calories
Cholesterol	<300 mg/day
Total calories	To achieve and maintain desirable weight
Step 2 diet	
Total fat	<30% of total calories
Saturated fatty acids	<7% of total calories
Polyunsaturated fatty acids	Up to 10% of total calories
Monounsaturated fatty acids	10–15% of total calories
Carbohydrates	50–60% of total calories
Protein	10–20% of total calories
Cholesterol	<200 mg/day
Total calories	To achieve and maintain desirable weight

In general, weight reduction affects VLDL levels more than LDL levels, so that patients with hypertriglyceridemia will respond better than those with hypercholesterolemia to weight reduction. Effects with diet change are normally seen within a few weeks, and lipid levels stabilize in a few months.

Recommended dietary modifications
Fish, chicken, turkey, and lean meats *Choose:* Fish, poultry without skin, lean cuts of beef, lamb, pork or veal; shellfish *Decrease:* Fatty cuts of beef, lamb, pork; spare ribs, organ meats, regular cold cuts, sausage, hot dogs, bacon, sardines, roe
Milk, cheese, yogurt, and dairy substitutes *Choose:* Skim or 1% fat milk (liquid, powdered, evaporated), buttermilk; non-fat or low-fat yogurt; low-fat cottage cheese (1 or 2% fat); low-fat cheeses; sherbet, sorbet *Decrease:* Whole milk (4% fat): regular, evaporated, condensed, cream, half and half, 2% milk, imitation milk products, most non-dairy creamers, whipped toppings; all natural cheeses, low-fat or 'light' sour cream, cream cheeses, sour cream; ice cream
Eggs *Choose:* Egg whites (two egg whites = one whole egg in recipes), cholesterol-free egg substitutes *Decrease:* Egg yolks
Fruits and vegetables *Choose:* Fresh, frozen, canned, or dried fruits and vegetables *Decrease:* Vegetables prepared in butter, cream, or other sauces
Breads and cereals *Choose:* Homemade baked goods using unsaturated oils sparingly, angel food cake, low-fat crackers, low-fat biscuits; rice, pasta; whole-grain breads and cereals *Decrease:* Commercial baked goods: pies, cakes, donuts, croissants, pastries, muffins, biscuits, high-fat crackers, high-fat cookies
Fats and oils *Choose:* Baking cocoa; unsaturated vegetable oils: corn, olive, rapeseed, safflower, sesame, soybean, sunflower; margarine or shortenings made from one of the unsaturated oils listed above, diet margarine; mayonnaise, salad dressings made with unsaturated oils listed above, low-fat dressings; seeds and nuts *Decrease:* Chocolate; butter, coconut oil, palm oil, palm kernel oil, lard, bacon fat; dressings made with egg yolk; coconut

15 Drug treatment

If diet, weight reduction, and exercise have not lowered total and LDL cholesterol levels to the desired ranges within 3 to 6 months, drug therapy should be considered.

▶ *Dietary management should continue even when drug therapy is administered since it will reduce the quantity of drug required. In fact, the dietary modifications made should continue as life-long habits.*

Five classes of lipid-lowering agents have been approved for use by the US Food and Drug Administration (FDA). The table below summarizes their application in the different hyperlipidemias, and on the following pages brief guidelines are given to their use in clinical practice.

Anion-exchange resins (bile acid sequestrants) (cholestyramine, colestipol): Reduce LDL cholesterol
Phenotype: II; *Genotypes*: Familal hypercholesterolemia, familial combined hyperlipidemia, polygenic hypercholesterolemia

---

Fibrates (gemfibrozil, clofibrate): Reduce serum triglycerides (also tend to reduce LDL cholesterol and moderately raise HDL cholesterol)
Phenotypes: IIb (gemfibrozil only), III, IV, V; *Genotypes*: Familial dysbetalipoproteinemia, familial hypertriglyceridemia, familial combined hyperlipidemia, familial type V hyperlipidemia

---

HMG CoA reductase inhibitors (lovastatin): Reduce LDL cholesterol (also moderately raise HDL cholesterol and reduce plasma triglycerides)
Phenotypes: IIa, IIb; *Genotypes*: Familial hypercholesterolemia, familial combined hyperlipidemia, polygenic hypercholesterolemia

---

Nicotinic acid: Reduces cholesterol and triglycerides (also markedly raises HDL cholesterol)
Phenotypes: IIa, IIb, III, IV, V; *Genotypes*: Familial hypercholesterolemia, familial combined hyperlipidemia, polygenic hypercholesterolemia, familial dysbetalipoproteinema, familial hypertriglyceridemia, familial type V hyperlipidemia

---

Probucol: Modestly reduces LDL cholesterol. (However, also lowers HDL cholesterol, sometimes markedly)
Phenotypes: IIa, IIb; *Genotypes*: Familial hypercholesterolemia, familial combined hyperlipidemia, polygenic hypercholesterolemia

---

BILE-ACID SEQUESTRANTS (anion-exchange resins: cholestyramine, colestipol)
First-line therapy for hypercholesterolemia. Effective in reducing LDL cholesterol (pure hypercholesterolemia).

Dosage: Starting dose is one packet twice daily (9 g packet cholestyramine, containing 4 g drug), increasing, if tolerated and necessary, to three packs twice daily.

Notes: **Constipation** is the major subjective side effect, overcome by bulking laxatives. Dosage may interfere with absorption of other drugs, which should be taken 1 to 3 hours before the dose of resin. Also, use may exacerbate **hypertriglyceridemia**. Diffuse gastrointestinal complaints such as **indigestion** are not uncommon.

Combinations: Can be combined with nicotinic acid.

Mechanism of action: Bind bile acids in the gut and abolish enterohepatic recirculation of bile acids, resulting in an increased need for cholesterol by the hepatocyte. More LDL receptors are then synthesized, increasing uptake of cholesterol by the liver, and thus lowering serum cholesterol concentrations.

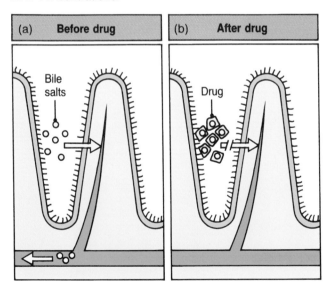

(a) Bile salts in the intestine are reabsorbed into the bloodstream. (b) Bile-acid sequestrants combine with bile salts and prevent this reabsorption.

NICOTINIC ACID (vitamin B$_3$)

First-line therapy for hypercholesterolemia. A broad-spectrum lipid-lowering drug, suitable for phenotypes IIa, IIb, III, IV and V. One of the few that lowers Lp(a) levels, and also raises HDL cholesterol by as much as 50%.

Dosage: 500 to 1500 mg three times daily. Dose may need to be increased in severe cases.

Notes: Gradually increasing the dose minimizes **flushing**, which can be further diminished in severe cases by indomethacin or aspirin. Raises **uric acid**, which should be monitored and treated if necessary. Can lead to **hepatitis**. Should be used with caution in patients with **peptic ulcer disease** or **diabetes**. Rare side effects include **acanthosis nigricans** and **retinal edema**, which disappears immediately on withdrawal.

Combinations: Can be combined with fibrates, cholestyramine, or HMG CoA reductase inhibitors, but combinations with the last-named drugs have been reported to increase slightly the risk of myopathy.

Mechanism of action: Unclear; diminishes VLDL synthesis and release from the liver.

HMG COA REDUCTASE INHIBITORS (lovastatin, fluvastatin*, pravastatin*, simvastatin*: *not approved by the FDA as of May 1990)

Useful in treating phenotypes IIa and IIb.

Dosage: Lovastatin, 20 to 40 mg once or twice daily.

Notes: Generally well tolerated. Serious side effects are so far few. Reversible **elevations of transaminase** and **creatine phosphokinase** are seen in a few patients.

Combinations: Combine very effectively with resins. In combination with fibrates or niacin results are good, but not recommended because of reported incidence of myositis.

Mechanism of action: Inhibit HMG CoA reductase, leading to increased expression of LDL receptors. This results in increased removal of LDL from the blood by the liver. LDL levels may also be lowered because of decreased production of LDL resulting from effects on VLDL synthesis.

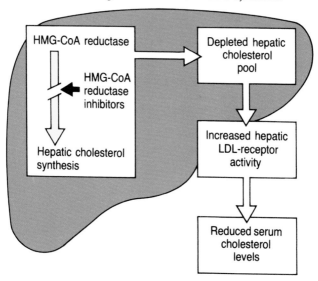

49

FIBRIC ACID DERIVATIVES (clofibrate, fenofibrate*, gemfibrozil: *not approved by the FDA as of May 1990)

Particularly effective in lowering VLDL, and thus in treating hypertriglyceridemia in phenotypes IIb, III, IV, and possibly V. Not all fibrates are compatible for all these phenotypes.

Dosage: Clofibrate, 2 g daily in divided doses; gemfibrozil, 1200 mg daily in divided doses.

Notes: Dosage is well tolerated, but transient **transaminase increases** are not infrequent. Rare side effects including **nausea**, **diarrhea**, **gallstones**, **alopecia**, and **muscle weakness** have been reported, with increases in **creatine kinase**. Clofibrate has been associated with an increased incidence of **gastrointestinal tumors**. Use with great caution when combined with HMG CoA reductase inhibitors, because of reports of increased incidence of myositis. May increase levels of LDL.

Combinations: Combinations with nicotinic acid and cholestyramine are well tolerated.

Mechanism of action: Mechanism of action is unclear. Possibilities include inhibition of lipolysis and stimulation of lipoprotein lipase synthesis.

PROBUCOL

In use as a cholesterol-lowering agent for more than 10 years. Effectively lowers LDL concentration by 20 to 30%, but also often lowers HDL cholesterol levels significantly. The clinical effect of the latter must be carefully evaluated. Useful in hypercholesterolemia of phenotypes IIa and IIb, and in the very rare homozygous familial hypercholesterolemia, where it may cause regression of xanthomas. Recent studies have suggested an antioxidative and antiatherosclerotic effect in Watanabe rabbits.

Dosage: 500 mg twice daily.

Notes: Serious side effects are so far few. An interesting property is its antioxidative action: it has been reported that probucol inhibits the oxidation of LDL and thereby renders LDL less attractive for the scavenger receptor of macrophages.

Mechanism of action: The mechanism whereby probucol lowers lipid levels is unknown.

16 Treatment of special groups

CHILDREN

Most pediatricians would agree that children with a family history of premature CHD should be screened for hypercholesterolemia. However, universal screening for children is still questioned by many pediatricians because of doubts about whether high childhood cholesterol levels are predictive of high levels in adulthood and about parents' potential over-reaction to dietary restrictions for the child [18].

Common-sense approaches to diet should be taught to preschoolers, especially to hyperlipidemic children. These include drinking low- or no-fat milk and avoiding fried foods. Additional dietary and drug treatment may be needed for children with severely elevated cholesterol levels and family histories of CHD. The NCEP currently suggests the use of bile-acid sequestrants for children with familial hypercholesterolemia. Additional guidelines are expected in the near future.

DIABETES MELLITUS

Various lipid abnormalities may occur in insulin-dependent diabetes. Optimal glycemic control should be achieved. In uncontrolled diabetes, triglycerides tend to be elevated, HDLs are often low, and LDLs may be high. However, diabetics may also have other causes of hyperlipidemia that need treatment.

In non–insulin-dependent diabetes, moderate hypertriglyceridemia, with or without hypercholesterolemia, and low HDL-cholesterol levels are common [19]. The development of renal complications aggravates these abnormalities. In addition to appropriate therapy for hyperglycemia, reduction of obesity helps decrease insulin resistance. Lipid-lowering therapy may be necessary if these methods fail.

HYPERTENSION

Hyperlipidemia is common in hypertensives. In this high-risk group, lipid-lowering drug therapy may be warranted if, despite dietary efforts, LDL cholesterol remains >160 mg/dL or total cholesterol remains >240 mg/dL. It is important to remember that some antihypertensive agents adversely influence serum lipids, particularly the beta blockers without intrinsic sympatho mimetic activity and thiazide diuretics, whereas alpha blockers, angiotensin converting enzyme inhibitors, and calcium antagonists do not [20].

RENAL IMPAIRMENT

The hyperlipidemia associated with renal impairment has been difficult to treat because most fibrates are secreted mainly in urine; therefore, the risk of side effects is greater. In renal failure VLDL is usually increased, whereas in nephrosis LDL is increased and VLDL may be also. It is likely that HMG CoA reductase inhibitors, some of which (fluvastatin, lovastatin, simvastatin) are excreted by the liver, will be used increasingly, especially in hypercholesterolemia secondary to the nephrotic syndrome. However, lovastatin must be used with great care in transplant patients receiving cyclosporine, since combined use has been reported to increase the risk of myopathy and rhabdomyolysis.

17 Radical therapy

▶ *Radical, that is non-pharmacological, methods should only be used if diet and drug therapy have failed to control hyperlipidemia or cannot be tolerated by the patient.*

PLASMA EXCHANGE
The chief indication for plasma exchange is **homozygous familial hypercholesterolemia**. It is well tolerated and remarkably free of side effects. However, it reduces not only LDL cholesterol but also HDL cholesterol. To be effective, it must be carried out repeatedly at 2- to 3-week intervals.

LDL APHERESIS
LDL apheresis involves diffusing plasma through adsorption columns that selectively bind LDL but not HDL. It must be carried out repeatedly at 2- to 3-week intervals.

PARTIAL ILEAL BYPASS
This procedure involves surgically bypassing the terminal one-third of the ileum. The main result is a 400% increase in bile acid excretion, which leads to an increased turnover of cholesterol to bile acids and a marked decrease in LDL cholesterol in plasma. Side effects can include diarrhea and renal stones.

Partial ileal bypass used to be administered to **heterozygous familial hypercholesterolemic** patients who did not tolerate bile-acid sequestrants. However, the use of HMG CoA reductase inhibitors, either alone or in combination with a small dose of a bile-acid sequestrant, has led to a decrease in the number of operations.

LIVER TRANSPLANTATION
The first successful transplantation of the liver from a normal donor into a homozygote for familial hypercholesterolemia was reported in 1984. Since then at least two other successful liver transplants have been reported. This operation represents the most definitive treatment for homozygous familial hypercholesterolemia currently available, but it is not without risk, including that associated with long-term administration of cyclosporine.

18 References

1. Schucker B, Wittes J, Cutler J, *et al.* Changes in physician perspectives on cholesterol and heart disease: results from two national surveys. *JAMA* 1987;258:3521–3526.

2. The Expert Panel. Report of the National Cholesterol Education Program Expert Panel on detection, evaluation, and treatment of high blood cholesterol in adults. *Arch Intern Med* 1988;148:36–69.

3. National Heart, Lung, and Blood Institute Consensus Development Panel. Treatment of hypertriglyceridemia. *JAMA* 1984;251:1196–1200.

4. Multiple Risk Factor Intervention Trial Research Group. Multiple Risk Factor Intervention Trial: Risk factor changes and mortality results. *JAMA* 1982;248:1465–1477.

5. Grundy SM, Vega GL. Causes of high blood cholesterol. *Circulation* 1990;81:412–427.

6. Grundy SM, Vega GL. Plasma cholesterol responsiveness to saturated fatty acids. *Am J Clin Nutr* 1988;47:822–824.

7. Keys A (ed). Coronary heart disease in seven countries. *Circulation* 1970;41(suppl I):I-1–I-211.

8. Anderson KM, Castelli WP, Levy D. Cholesterol and mortality. 30 years of follow-up from the Framingham Study. *JAMA* 1987;257:2176–2180.

9. Brensike JF, Levy RI, Kelsey SK, *et al.* Effects of therapy with cholestyramine on progression of coronary arteriosclerosis: Results of the NHLBI Type II Coronary Intervention Study. *Circulation.* 1984;69:313–324.

10. Blankenhorn DH, Nessim SA, Johnson RL, Sanmarco ME, Azen SP, Cashin-Hemphill L. Beneficial effects of combined colestipol-niacin therapy on coronary atherosclerosis and coronary venous bypass grafts. *JAMA* 1987;257:3233–3240.

11. Brown BG, Lin JT, Schaefer SM, *et al.* Niacin or lovastatin, combined with colestipol, regress coronary atherosclerosis and prevent clinical events in men with elevated apolipoprotein B. *Circulation.* 1989;80(suppl II):II-266.

12. Lipid Research Clinics Program. The Lipid Research Clinics Coronary Primary Prevention Trial results. I. Reduction in incidence of coronary heart disease. *JAMA* 1984;251:351–364.

13. Mannienen V, Elo O, Frick MH, *et al.* Lipid alterations and decline in the incidence of coronary heart disease in the Helsinki Heart Study. *JAMA* 1988;260:641–651.

14. Canner PL, Berge KG, Wenger NK, *et al.* Fifteen year mortality in Coronary Drug Project patients: Long-term benefit with niacin. *J Am Coll Cardiol* 1986;8:1245–1255.

15. Hjermann I, Holme I, Leren P. Oslo Study Diet and Antismoking Trial. Results after 102 months. *Am J Med* 1986;80:7–11.

16. Carlson LA, Rosenhamer G. Reduction of mortality in the Stockholm Ischaemic Heart Disease Secondary Prevention study by combined treatment with clofibrate and nicotinic acid. *Acta Med Scand* 1988;223:405–418.

17. National Cholesterol Education Program. Current status of blood cholesterol measurement in clinical laboratories in the United States. *NIH Publication No. 88-2928,* 1988.

18. American Academy of Pediatrics Committee on Nutrition. Indications for cholesterol testing in children. *Pediatrics* 1989;83:141–142.

19. Reaven GM. Insulin resistance and the development of cardiovascular disease. *Clinician* 1989;7:10–14.

20. 1988 Report of the Joint National Committee on Detection, Evaluation, and Treatment of High Blood Pressure. *Arch Intern Med* 1988;148:1023–1038.

Subject index